PREGNANCY NUTRITION

A Great Start for Baby

Garry Wainscott M.Hlth.Sc. (Human Nutrition)

Disclaimer

The material in this publication is of the nature of general comment only
and does not represent medical or professional advice. It is not intended
to provide specific guidance for particular circumstances, and it should not
be relied on as the basis for any decision to take action or not take action
on any matter it covers. Readers should obtain professional advice where
appropriate before making any such decision. To the maximum extent
permitted by law, the author disclaims all responsibility and liability to any
person, arising directly or indirectly from any person taking or not taking
action based on the information in this publication.

Pregnancy Nutrition — A Great Start for Baby
© 2014 by Garry Wainscott
Perth, Western Australia

ISBN-13: 978-1499745115
ISBN 10: 1499745117
Library of Congress Control Number: 2014910131
CreateSpace Independent Publishing Platform
North Charleston, South Carolina

CONTENTS

ABOUT THE AUTHOR

Garry Wainscott, born in New Zealand, is a pharmacist by trade and dispensed both human and veterinary treatments before moving into the pharmaceutical industry. After eight years with the first company he worked for, he became a key manager with a major US-based international company involved both in pharmaceuticals and in nutrition products. Eventually, Garry was promoted to a general management position.

After nine years in New Zealand with the international company, he transferred to Asian postings, living and working in Indonesia, Singapore, and Thailand in key marketing roles and general management. He spent twenty-six years managing operations both in Southeast Asia and South Asia before retiring to start his own business, TeknoLink Nutrition, based in Perth, Western Australia.

Garry's involvement with human nutrition began in 1967, initially in infant nutrition. Then he began specializing in sports nutrition. He planned dietary intake for ultra-long-distance runners and provided protein supplements to swimmers, athletes (including key New Zealand Olympic medal-winning middle-distance runners), and various national sports teams. He later became involved with child, maternal, and geriatric dietary supplements.

While domiciled in Singapore, Garry served as president of the Singapore Association of Pharmaceutical Industries (SAPI) and chairman of the Advertising Standards Authority of Singapore (ASAS). In 1983, he founded the Singapore Nutrition and Dietetics Association (SNDA).

From 2003 to 2006, Garry lectured on various infant-nutrition topics to pædiatricians at various venues in Malaysia, Indonesia, Sri Lanka, the Philippines, China, Hong Kong, and Taiwan. He was a guest speaker at the 2005 Obstetrics & Gynaecology of Singapore Congress and a guest speaker at the 2006 Obstetrical & Gynaecology Society of Malaysia Congress.

Garry graduated from Deakin University, Australia, with a Graduate Diploma in Human Nutrition and a Master of Health Science (Human Nutrition) degree.

ACKNOWLEDGMENTS

Special thanks go to Lily Withers, my joint-venture partner, for her insights that relate to potential readers of this book. She discerned the information gap for "mums-to-be" who are keen to know what they need to do with their nutrition prior to conception and throughout their pregnancy to provide their babies with the best possible start to life. The gap lies between food lists and recipes on the one hand and the superficial information and "old wives' tales" on the other. Filling that gap requires up-to-date knowledge of important information from reliable sources on particular nutrients.

A book to help fill that gap requires a background of decades of persistent updating of information as science makes steady progress on so many issues. The sources of this information from so many medical and nutritional specialists over that period of time are too numerous to list. However, I would like to extend my special appreciation to Professor Alexandra McManus, Director of the Centre of Excellence for Science, Seafood, and Health, Curtin University, Perth, Western Australia, who so readily and kindly provided me with the most recent information on the importance of maternal seafood-derived Omega-3 to the brain development of babies in the womb.

PREFACE

Many books provide cooking recipes for pregnancy. This book is definitely not one of those.

Rather than the old "Grandma told Mother, and Mother told me" pathway that helped mothers-to-be do at least some of the right things for Baby, this book sets out to put into some understandable form the up-to-date, science-based information that can help give your baby a better start in life.

This book provides evidence-based insight into key nutrients that have the ability to make a difference to both the health and the development of the fœtus (the baby in the womb). This information should give the new baby a good base from which to benefit from breast-feeding or, if or when necessary, the feeding of a quality baby formula.

Ideally, a pregnancy should be planned well in advance. Many nutrients should be in plentiful levels within a woman's body well before she realizes that the pregnancy is indeed a fact. Folate is one of those; iron is another.

During fœtal development, it is important that key nutrient levels are maintained at all times. For example, brain growth is time-dependent. Different developmental processes occur at specific chronological ages, and once the time for a phase of growth has passed, it cannot be restarted. There is no "rewind" mechanism that can be used to recover opportunities missed.

Weight management during pregnancy is also important, both for mothers and for the fœtal development of the child-to-be.

The information within this book also covers many nonnutrient-related lifestyle factors that should be addressed.

EXPECTING THE "EXPECTING"

The period of pregnancy is often referred to as "expecting" (i.e., "expecting" to have a new baby soon). Ideally, when planning a pregnancy, the period of expecting should start much earlier than conception. Often, the intended mother-to-be may need to make lifestyle changes to improve her health status so that she can provide the best environment for her future baby's well-being.

Good nutrition is important at an early stage for the baby's brain growth and development. Certain nutrients exert their effects within a narrow window quite soon after conception. Brain development is a process that unfolds over time. Thus, the timing of developmental events is critical. There are multiple levels of timing, and each plays an important role in shaping the developing brain. Once the time for a particular phase of brain growth has passed, it cannot be restarted.

For example, later in this book, I discuss the importance of a mother's folate adequacy for the proper development of her baby, to avoid *spina bifida* and its severe consequences. Spina bifida occurs when, as a result of a deficiency in the mother's available folate, the neural tube of the fœtus fails to close properly, leaving the spinal cord exposed. The closure of the neural tube should take place about twenty-three days after conception. However, a significant number of women do not realize they are pregnant until twenty-one to twenty-eight days after conception. That is too late to start folate supplementation as a means of avoiding spina bifida.

Past recommendations have been to begin folate supplementation about one month before conception to enable a progressive improvement in folate status within the mother's body by the time of conception. But research carried out at the Nutrition Department, University of Otago, Dunedin, New Zealand, several years ago found more satisfactory folate levels in those mothers who began folate supplementation *three* months before conception.

A more recent study (2012) conducted in Australia provided evidence that folic-acid supplements taken before pregnancy and possibly ongoing through pregnancy may protect against childhood brain tumours.

Other nutrients whose deficiency at the time of conception may damage brain growth and development are selenium and vitamin A. Later supplementation with these nutrients will do little to alter damage that may have taken place during the first twelve weeks after conception. Additional nutrients that play an ongoing role in brain development throughout pregnancy include protein, iron, zinc, and iodine.

A mother-to-be should visit her doctor as early as possible to obtain blood tests to determine levels of such important baby-development nutrients as iron and vitamin D. In many populations, iron and vitamin D deficiencies are extremely common. Included in blood testing should be the T4 (thyroxine) test for thyroid function. Even moderately low T4 levels in the mother may be damaging to the developing fœtus. Research published in 2012 in Australia shows that the average iodine intake of Australian women fell short of recommended levels, despite local laws in 2009 mandating the iodine fortification of bread. This trend has prompted endocrinologists to call for universal thyroid screening of all pregnant women.

Severe weight loss as a result of dieting during the last two trimesters of pregnancy may be at the expense of the baby's growth and development. I discourage it because it can cause restricted intake of important nutrients and, as a result, may cause fœtal stunting. For this reason, any weight-reduction programs that may be necessary should be carried out well before conception is planned.

Intended mothers who smoke cigarettes need to ask themselves, "Is it really worth the risk?" This applies equally to the mother's heath and to the well-being of the fœtus, infant, and child. Researchers at the University of Otago in Dunedin, New Zealand, have shed new light on the reason why mothers who smoke during pregnancy — particularly during the later stages of pregnancy — tend to have babies with lower birth weights and serious complications. They found severe DNA damage to the cells in the placenta of mothers who smoked during pregnancy. Such damage to the placental cells is likely to interfere with the transfer of adequate nutrients from mother to unborn child. It also can interfere with important hormone production within the placenta. The researchers identified greatly increased rates of double-strand DNA breaks (a severe form of DNA damage) in the placental cells of smoking mothers.

Lower birth weight is not the only negative factor associated with smoking during pregnancy. Higher rates of miscarriage, preterm births, difficulty during childbirth, sudden infant death syndrome (SIDS), asthma, and glue ear all have been associated with smoking during pregnancy.

"Secondary smoking" — the close presence of spouses, relatives, or friends who smoke — also may be harmful and therefore should be avoided. A close association between cigarette smoking and breast cancer and cervical cancer and a close association between cigarette smoking and lung cancer or later emphysema also have been documented. These medical facts should be sufficient to encourage mothers-to-be to cease smoking and to commit to not resuming smoking for the remainder of their lives.

Substance abuse should be halted many months before conception and throughout conception. A 2012 study of more than three thousand Australian and New Zealand pregnant women found that marijuana use prior to pregnancy was the second-highest risk factor for premature birth in women who smoked marijuana. These mothers were 2.5 times more likely to deliver preterm than nonsmokers. There were also concerns about the effect of THC (the active ingredient in marijuana) on the fœtus's brain.

Most "recreational" drugs affect chemical pathways within the brain. With regular use of these drugs, those affected pathways may never totally resume normal function. The brain of a fœtus grows at a rapid rate, so it makes sense that during this rapid development period, a baby's brain should not be exposed to such substances that cross the blood/brain barrier. In addition to avoiding recreational drugs throughout the periods of pregnancy and breast-feeding, prospective mothers would be wise to avoid such drugs during the weeks prior to conception so that no residual drugs remain in their bodies.

Alcohol consumption should be avoided altogether during the period of pregnancy. Alcohol can cross the placenta so that the blood alcohol level in the fœtus quickly rises to the same blood-alcohol level as in the mother. Any harm to the unborn baby from these blood-alcohol levels can take place at any stage during pregnancy. Further, any resulting harm to development and behaviour can last well beyond childhood into adult life.

For pregnancy, there is no "safe limit" for alcohol consumption. The risk involved with alcohol consumption during pregnancy lies with what is referred to as "fœtal alcohol syndrome" or "fœtal alcohol spectrum disorder" (FASD). This is a general term for the various adverse effects caused by exposure to alcohol during pregnancy, such as alcohol-related neurodevelopmental disorders, alcohol-related birth defects, growth retardation, and facial anomalies. FASD may include postnatal growth deficiency (lack of catch-up growth after the baby is born, despite good nutrition), central nervous system abnormalities and dysfunction, developmental delays, mental retardation, heart murmur, and learning and behavioural disorders.

Risk to the fœtus has been demonstrated to occur even from moderate levels of alcohol consumption during pregnancy, including occasional binge drinking. Increased risk of child behaviour problems, developmental delays, and intellectual disability results from exposure during pregnancy at even moderate (three to four standard drinks per occasion) or higher levels of consumption, especially during the second half of pregnancy.

For the woman who enjoys her Sauvignon Blanc, Pinot Noir, or Brut Champagne, for the well-being of the new life she is bringing into this world, the total avoidance of alcohol should not be too much of a hardship to endure for the nine months of the pregnancy and also perhaps for the first few months of breast-feeding.

Here is another "sobering" thought for consideration: Generally, approximately half of all pregnancies are unplanned. Awareness of pregnancy may not take place until the sixth week after conception or perhaps even later — yet the fœtus is more vulnerable to the effects of alcohol during early pregnancy, with high risk between two and eight weeks after conception. Therefore, it makes much sense when planning a pregnancy to avoid high consumption of alcohol or binge drinking as soon as pregnancy planning commences.

If you are in the habit of saying, "And I'll have fries with that," then pregnancy is a time when you might want to ease off on the consumption of french fries and potato chips. When starch-rich foods such as potatoes are cooked at high temperatures (e.g., frying or baking), a substance known as "acrylamide" is formed. Scientists who carried out a study published in the journal *Environmental Health Perspectives* in 2012 reported that women who had a high intake of acrylamide during pregnancy were more likely to have small babies with lower birth weights and smaller head circumferences than women who had low dietary exposure to acrylamide.

In the past, such physical outcomes have been associated with slower neurodevelopment and adverse health effects early in life.

Talking about "and I'll have fries with that" raises a new issue. It is my personal contention that there is no such thing as "junk food" — only "junk diets." Eaten in moderation, most foods can be quite acceptable. It is when the so-called "junk foods" become a frequent and regular part of the diet that they become "junk diets." In March 2013 in *The FASEB Journal* (Federation of the American Societies for Experimental Biology), researchers discussed a study that revealed that frequent consumption of "junk foods" during pregnancy and lactation influences a preference in the offspring for these foods later in life. This study was done in rats because, for ethical reasons, it could not be done in humans. The researchers found that maternal "junk-food" diets resulted in changes in the opioid receptors within the reward pathway of the brain. They suggested that subsequent desensitization may explain the preference for "junk food" in offspring.

Healthy nutrition should be well established before pregnancy, for the benefit of both mother and child. A report published in the *British Journal of Psychiatry* in October 2013 outlined a study in the United Kingdom. Researchers assessed 6,979 mother-and-child pairs for maternal depression symptoms five times between eighteen weeks of pregnancy and when their children were thirty-three months (almost three years) old. The researchers found that a higher level of depressive symptoms was related to lower levels of healthy nutrition and higher levels of unhealthy nutrition. There was a similar relationship to the level of cognition in their children. The researchers concluded that healthy nutrition should be started before pregnancy to reduce the likelihood of both prenatal and postnatal depression in mothers and for healthy development of their children.

If you are a heavy coffee drinker, it could be beneficial to ease off the frequency of those cups of coffee. A Norwegian study published in *BMC Medicine* in February 2013 found that maternal caffeine consumption was related to low-birth-weight babies. If you drink "high energy" or sports drinks containing caffeine often, it could be a wise decision to reduce consumption throughout your pregnancy.

And, when you are "expecting," there are many factors besides nutrition to consider. For example, recent increases have been noted in the frequency of pertussis ("whooping cough") cases in babies, as well as deaths associated with this infection. If you did not have a pertussis vaccination prior to conception, it is wise to consult your doctor to seek advice on this vaccination between the twenty-eighth and thirty-eighth weeks of pregnancy.

BABY, YOU, AND MAYBE GRANDMA, TOO?

Soon after your baby is born, it will be natural for you to watch the development of features, trying to find those that reflect your own features and those that reflect the father's features. What will not be so visible are those inner-body "features" such as appropriate heart development, liver and kidney function, hormonal influences, brain development, and many other contributions to the present and future health of your baby.

Science continues to seek to determine which factors influence a baby's future health and well-being, not only while the baby is in its mother's womb and in babyhood and early childhood, but also during the mother's prepregnancy. The environment the baby's mother—and even the baby's maternal grandmother—lived in while growing up have an impact on a baby's well-being. Dr. David Barker, a physician and epidemiologist at the University of Southampton, UK, noted that "the mother is the product of her lifetime nutrition—and even her own mother's nutrition, too, because most or all of her eggs are formed before birth."

11

It really started in the late 1980s with observations by Dr. Barker that babies whose birth weight was lower than normal were more likely in adult life to die from heart disease. His publication, in 1992, of his findings from birth and death certificates of thousands of Hertfordshire (UK) residents generated a great deal of interest in the phenomenon. In 1995, the *British Medical Journal* named this theory the "Barker Hypothesis," and it formed the nucleus of further international studies.

The early focus was on the observation that smaller babies tended to be a reflection of poor nourishment within the womb or from high stress levels in the mother. More recently, animal studies have demonstrated that a poor flow of nutrients across the placenta causes the fœtus's body to respond by attempting to form organs with the nutrients that are available. This results in fewer muscle cells in the heart, less skeletal muscle in the limbs, fewer insulin-producing cells in the pancreas, and fewer nephrons in the kidneys for filtering urine.

Of course, the nutritional state of the mother during prepregnancy and throughout pregnancy also may play a role in restricting nutrient availability to the fœtus. This was an influential factor in babies born during and after the severe food restrictions during World War II, and it continues today in underdeveloped nations with high rates of malnutrition. However, even in developed nations, poor eating habits, an unbalanced diet, and a mother's body composition can exert influences on the health and development of a baby, not only in the early stages of life, but into adulthood.

The ongoing studies, many of which are now exploring the influence of the fœtal environment and nutrition on health in later life, are focusing on subtle changes in DNA. It will take many years to reach conclusions. Meanwhile, good care and good nutrition throughout pregnancy are important in giving babies their best start in life.

This book reviews many of the key nutrients that are needed to provide your baby with adequacy for development.

EATING FOR TWO?

"Eating for two" does *not* mean "a Big Mac and fries for me and another Big Mac and fries for Baby." Instead, it means eating healthily and appropriately for the well-being of both the mother, whose body is undergoing significant changes after conception, and the fœtus, which starts out as a single cell at conception but is still, sixteen weeks later, only about one-quarter of 1 percent its mother's weight. That is, the fœtus is four hundred times less in weight than its mother.

Conception is a signal to the mother's body to prepare for the pregnancy, and this largely takes place under the influence of hormonal changes. By about the tenth day after fertilization of the ovum (egg), the embryo becomes embedded in the wall of the uterus and the placenta, which will transport nutrients and oxygen from the mother to the fœtus over the months ahead, begins to form. Immediately, the placenta begins to secrete hormones that influence the development of the pregnancy. Various placental hormones promote breast development; stimulate uterine growth to accommodate the growing fœtus; and regulate maternal glucose, protein, and fat levels to ensure that these are always available to the fœtus.

In April 2013, the medical journal *Pediatric Obesity* published the results of a study that found that mothers with excessive weight gain during pregnancy had babies (measured within seventy-two hours of birth) with greater body fat. It was considered that this increased *adiposity* (the amount of fat in the fatty tissues) at birth may predispose these children to increased risk of obesity. It also highlights the impact of mothers gaining excess weight during pregnancy.

Early "eating for two" also may play a part in increasing the degree of adiposity in newborns. In August 2013, the US medical journal *Obstetrics & Gynecology* published a study that outlined the importance of the timing of excessive weight gain as a factor influencing the elevation of body fat in newborns. The researchers found that the babies of women who gained weight excessively during the first half of pregnancy had a greater risk of newborn adiposity than those women who had a total excessive weight gain over the entire pregnancy. The researchers concluded that "prevention of early excessive weight gain should be encouraged in the period before conception and reinforced early in pregnancy."

During pregnancy, an appropriate weight gain by the mother (single-baby pregnancy) is characterized by these guidelines:

- 1.2 kg (2 lb., 10 oz.) of increased blood volume

- 1.2 kg (2 lb., 10 oz.) of increased extracellular water within the body

- 4.0 kg (8 lb., 13 oz.) of additional body fat

- 0.4 kg (14 oz.) of increased breast tissue

- 0.7 kg (1 lb., 9 oz.) of placenta tissue

- 0.9 kg (2 lb.) of the amniotic fluid in which the fœtus is bathed

- 0.9 kg (2 lb.) of increased tissue in the uterus

- 3.3 kg (7 lb., 4 oz.) the weight of the full-term baby

This represents a total gain in weight of 12.6 kg (27 lb., 12 oz.), requiring increased nutritional intake by the mother. This is regarded as a healthy weight gain for a single-baby pregnancy, and pregnant women should make an effort to avoid weight gain in excess of that level.

Excessive weight gain during pregnancy is now considered to make a significant contribution to the "obesity epidemic" currently evident in so many countries around the world. A study of 41,133 mothers and their children in Arkansas, USA, published in October 2013, found that the risk of obesity in the children up to twelve years of age increased when their mothers had excessive weight gain during their pregnancy. Apparently, the effect of maternal weight gain during pregnancy continues through their children's childhoods. The study found that one in twelve children born to women who gained 40 lb. (18.2 kg) or more during their pregnancy had an increased likelihood of childhood obesity.

Even if there has been no medical history of diabetes, a condition known as *gestational diabetes* can occur during pregnancy. This is a relatively common condition during pregnancy and is usually a consequence of the altered hormonal balance at this time. The fœtus can use only glucose to meet its energy needs. Therefore, maternal metabolism is keyed to making sure that adequate amounts of glucose are supplied to meet the requirements of the fœtus.

Pregnant women have normal insulin responses to glucose early in pregnancy, but in the later months it takes more insulin to remove the same amount of glucose from the blood. The reasons remain unclear, but hormonal interactions are considered a likely factor. It is thought that the presence of human placental lactogen may interfere with susceptible insulin receptors, thus making the reduction of blood-sugar levels less efficient.

Gestational diabetes has an incidence of 3 to 10 percent of all pregnancies in general populations, with the incidence in Asia thought to be at the higher end of this range. It is believed that with more thorough screening of pregnant women, the incidence would be around 8 percent (about one in twelve) of pregnancies. Mothers who are overweight or have a family history of diabetes mellitus are at greater risk of developing gestational diabetes.

At the 2012 meeting of the European Association for the Study of Diabetes, research results were presented indicating a significant link between vitamin D deficiency during the first three months of pregnancy and an increased likelihood of developing gestational diabetes. A further European study is now being conducted to determine whether supplementation with vitamin D may prevent gestational diabetes.

A healthy lifestyle that includes eating a healthy diet, controlling weight, and getting regular exercise prior to pregnancy lessens a woman's risk of getting gestational diabetes. Such a healthy lifestyle also should be maintained throughout the pregnancy. Any additional nutritional intake for maintaining adequate energy levels during pregnancy should have a low glycæmic index (GI) to avoid exacerbating an underlying condition.

In December 2013, a commentary from the University of Adelaide, Australia, appearing in *Evidence-Based Nursing*, published by the British Medical Journal Publishing Group, noted that a number of research teams around the world are showing that consumption of a lot of red meat and processed meats appears to be linked with a significant risk of developing gestational diabetes. Even high consumption of red meat and processed meats prior to becoming pregnant appears to increase the risk of gestational diabetes. Consumption of fish or poultry does not seem to have that effect. Before and during pregnancy, only modest amounts of red meat should be consumed and, instead, eating more vegetables and nonmeat protein (e.g., a small serving of nuts each day) is recommended.

It is important that you discuss with your doctor a program for oral glucose tolerance testing (OGTT) during pregnancy. It is usual for testing to take place between weeks twenty-four and twenty-eight of pregnancy. However, if you have a history of gestational diabetes in a previous pregnancy or a family history of type 2 diabetes, or if you are overweight, then your doctor may recommend oral glucose tolerance testing earlier in the pregnancy.

In most cases, gestational diabetes does not continue following the birth of the baby. However, an increased risk of developing type 2 diabetes later in life exists.

Although childhood attention-deficit/hyperactivity disorder (ADHD) may have associations with heredity and environment, two studies published in medical journals in 2012 also found a significant relationship between gestational diabetes and ADHD. To help reduce the likelihood of developing gestational diabetes during pregnancy, it is wise to implement a healthy eating program that includes the following steps:

- Maintaining a healthy weight by increasing energy intake by no more than is required for the daily needs of your own changing body and the growth stage of your developing baby

- Avoiding sugar (sucrose)-laden drinks and sodas. Nutritionists and dietitians regard refined sugar (sucrose) as "empty calories" because it provides no required nutrients — just extra, non-useful calories.

- Eating your fruit as "fruit" instead of consuming large volumes of fruit juices, which have high sugar content

If you develop gestational diabetes, it is wise to see a dietitian to obtain expert advice about a modified diet. He or she probably will make recommendations like the following:

- Eat small amounts on a frequent basis rather than large, single meals.

- Avoid carbohydrates in the form of sugar, and instead eat those that are less likely to cause rapid blood glucose increases, such as multigrain breads, pasta, lentils, and beans.

- Reduce, and preferably avoid, the intake of potatoes and white rice. If some rice is required, then the lower-GI Basmati or Doongara types of rice are preferable.

- Monitor body-weight increases closely.

MORE PROTEIN

It is estimated that 925 g (2 lb.) of protein is deposited during a pregnancy involving 12.6 kg (27 lb., 12 oz.) of maternal weight gain and an infant weighing 3.3 kg (7 lb., 4 oz.) at birth.

Studies suggest that relatively more protein may be stored during early pregnancy — perhaps in skeletal muscle — and then mobilized at later stages of pregnancy. In addition to deposition of protein nitrogen throughout pregnancy, protein *turnover* is increased by the twelfth week of pregnancy; it remains high in the second trimester and is the same or lower in the third trimester. Consequently, increased protein needs during pregnancy may be more uniform than earlier estimates indicated.

Much of the daily protein requirements of the human body are met by "recycling." What most people don't realize is that most proteins in our bodies are replaced every few days — even in cells that divide rarely, such as those in the liver and nervous system. And different proteins are degraded at widely differing rates. Some have half-lives as short as twenty minutes, whereas others within the same cell may last for days or weeks.

"Recycling" even occurs within the gut as the enzymes (yes, enzymes are proteins) that digest our food, and also the cells lining our intestines, which are replaced every three to five days, are themselves "digested" to have their protein broken down into component amino acids. That enables the body to build completely new proteins from those amino acids.

In addition to this "recycling," the recommended daily intake of quality protein from the diet for nonpregnant women of child-bearing age is 46 g (1.6 oz.) per day. In pregnancy, the efficiency (~70 percent) with which dietary protein is converted to fœtal, placental, and maternal tissues needs to be taken into account when estimating the increase in daily intake of dietary protein of 25 g (0.9 oz,) per day that is required during the second and third trimesters of pregnancy.

With the recommended daily dietary intake for protein for nonpregnant women of child-bearing age at 46 g of quality protein per day, an incremental dietary intake of 25 g of quality protein per day represents a rather significant 54 percent increase in total dietary protein intake in pregnant women — and this presumes that a woman already was taking the full recommended daily intake for nonpregnant women.

Often, many pregnant women find it difficult to increase the amount of protein they eat in normal meals or to eat additional meals containing sufficient high-quality protein. In those cases, a high-protein dietary supplement may be required to augment their food intake.

Dairy milk and/or milk-based protein supplements are a good source of quality protein. Later in pregnancy, there is greater use of muscles, and high muscle usage can cause more rapid break-down of the *branched-chain amino acids* (BCAAs), which are prevalent in muscle tissue. The human body cannot manufacture these BCAAs (leucine, isoleucine, and valine), so they must be replenished from the diet. With 21 percent of the protein in dairy milk in the form of these BCAA, it is a good dietary protein you can use to increase your daily protein intake.

"Raw" milk should not be consumed during pregnancy. It presents a realistic and unnecessary threat because of its possible contamination with pathogenic bacteria such as *Campylobacter*, *Salmonella*, and *E. coli*, which can cause serious health consequences. Drink or use only cow's milk that has been pasteurized (heat-treated). Recent research has confirmed that pasteurization does not destroy the nutritional and health benefits of milk.

THE IMPORTANCE OF IRON

Iron is an essential element for the viability of body cells and for cell proliferation. It is also an essential component of the proteins that are involved in energy metabolism. The body's major requirement for iron is for the production of the hæmoglobin in the red blood cells.

In pregnancy, the body needs iron to replace the usual basal losses. This allows expansion of the red-cell mass as the mother's blood volume increases and provides iron to the fœtus and placenta. It also enables the body to store iron to be able to replace the blood lost during delivery.

It is estimated that the total iron needed for a pregnancy is approximately 1,040 mg. Of that amount, 840 mg is lost from the body permanently, and 200 mg is retained to act as a reservoir of iron when blood volume decreases after delivery. Similar estimates give a requirement for an additional 1,200 g of iron required *before* pregnancy to prevent the development of pregnancy-related iron deficiency.

There is little need for increased iron intake during the first trimester (first three months) of pregnancy because the cessation of iron loss from menstruation is compensatory for the small requirements during the early part of pregnancy. However, the extra 1,000 mg is required during the second and third trimesters of pregnancy to meet the needs of a normal pregnancy.

As well as the presence of iron in the hæmoglobin of the red blood cells and in specific enzymes, the body has the ability to store iron. The incremental (additional) amount of "storage" iron required due to pregnancy is about 550 mg. This is greater than the stores of most women, which seldom exceed 500 mg, and are more typically in the 100 mg range. That amount is even less than 100 mg in a considerable number of women.

The requirement for extra iron during pregnancy usually exceeds the amount that most women's bodies can absorb from a good diet. Therefore, iron needs to be provided mainly from other external sources, and in most cases, it will come in the form of iron supplements.

In the third trimester, there is a natural increase in the proportion of iron that is absorbed from dietary sources. While this may be adequate for well-nourished mothers with an already high iron status, in most pregnancies and especially in regions of iron undernutrition, women need iron supplementation. Iron undernutrition is endemic in most areas throughout Asia.

You will recall from "*Eating for Two?*" that approximately 1.2 kg (2 lb., 10 oz.) of the weight gain during pregnancy is attributed to increased blood volume. "Low" hæmoglobin is the most common nutritional biochemical problem encountered in everyday prenatal care.

Iron-deficiency anæmia during pregnancy may compromise delivery of oxygen to the fœtus. An anæmic woman is less able to tolerate obstetric complications during childbirth than a woman who is not anæmic. Obvious iron-deficiency anæmia is a late-stage indication of a significant lack of iron, and there are two earlier stages of iron malnutrition as well. The three stages are as follows:

- Stage 1: Iron depletion

- Stage 2: Iron deficiency without anæmia

- Stage 3: Iron deficiency with anæmia

Even at Stage 1, iron depletion during pregnancy can have adverse effects on the development of the fœtus and the baby after birth. However, it is only at Stage 3 that iron depletion becomes clinically evident. It is for this reason that both before pregnancy and during pregnancy, a pregnant woman should be under the guidance of her doctor for blood testing for iron status and, when appropriate, iron therapy to improve iron status. Do not be tempted to self-medicate. Although at least one hundred oral iron products are available in retail outlets, fewer than six contain adequate amounts of elemental iron that can treat iron deficiency successfully. Even with a supplement, it can take three to six months to replenish lost iron stores fully.

Often it is considered that iron supplementation during pregnancy may be a cause of constipation. Constipation is not uncommon during pregnancy, probably due to dietary changes, hormonal changes, and metabolic changes. During constipation, it is wise to observe stools that are eventually passed. If iron supplements are being taken, excess iron that is not being absorbed into the body will cause dark coloration of the stools. For that reason, it is tempting to suggest that there is a link between iron supplementation and constipation, but that has not been demonstrated scientifically. More recent studies suggest that iron absorption by the body is better when supplements are taken every second day rather than every day. Iron absorption is also better when it is taken between meals, preferably on an empty stomach, rather than at the same time as meals.

Iron stores are built up in the fœtus during the last few weeks of pregnancy. It is important that a baby is born with good iron stores from maternal provision during the last trimester (three months) of pregnancy. If a baby becomes anæmic (iron deficient) during the first few months following birth, it can give rise to significantly lower mental and motor test scores later in childhood. Even with iron therapy to correct the anæmia in babyhood, it is often insufficient to reverse behavioural and developmental disturbances later in babyhood and in childhood. Studies have clearly demonstrated that even at eleven to fourteen years of age, those who were severely iron deficient early in babyhood scored lower on measures of mental and motor functioning than did children who had good iron status during babyhood.

New evidence suggests that the poorer cognitive motor skills (for example, coordination), and social/emotional outcomes caused by iron deficiency during babyhood have longer-term consequences, even into adulthood. An internationally renowned researcher on the impact of iron deficiency, Betsy Lozoff, recently completed a twenty-five-year follow-up study on babies who were chronically iron deficient, and received iron therapy for three months. The results of this study, published in *The Journal of Pediatrics* in 2013, revealed that, despite using iron therapy to treat their iron deficiency in babyhood, these adults, on average, completed one year less of schooling and were less likely to complete secondary school, go on to further education and training, or get married. Further, their emotional health was rated worse, and more negative emotions and detachment/dissociation were reported.

This latest study once again emphasizes that a good iron status needs to be maintained throughout pregnancy and into breast-feeding for the long-term development and well-being of your baby through childhood and adulthood. It is important to take steps to avoid iron deficiency in your baby. Once iron deficiency is present in babyhood, iron therapy is unlikely to reverse all of the missed opportunities lost from delayed development.

Iron deficiency in babyhood potentially affects developmental brain processes, including myelination, energy metabolism, and hippocampal growth, most of which are dependent on iron-containing hæmoproteins or iron-sulphur compounds that are adversely affected by iron deficiency.

Brain growth is time-dependent. Different developmental processes occur at specific chronological ages, and once the time for a phase of growth has passed, it cannot be restarted. For this reason, a healthy iron level is important for the mother before and during pregnancy and also during breast-feeding for the benefit of her baby over the years ahead.

GETTING ENOUGH VITAMIN D

Community-based studies have shown that the incidence of vitamin D deficiency in pregnancy is quite high.

In "*Eating for Two?*" I mentioned that research results have indicated a significant link between vitamin D deficiency during the first three months of pregnancy and an increased likelihood of developing gestational diabetes.

Recent nutrition research has highlighted the need for mothers to have good levels of vitamin D in the body throughout pregnancy, not only for themselves but also for their babies. Low levels of vitamin D during pregnancy are now believed to have adverse effects on birth outcomes, as well as later, upon the ongoing development in the children of those mothers.

In 2012, the prestigious medical journal *Pediatrics* (American Academy of Pediatrics) published a Spanish study suggesting that vitamin D deficiency during pregnancy could hinder babies' brain and motor development. The researchers measured maternal vitamin D levels during pregnancy. Then, when the babies were fourteen months of age, psychologists assessed their mental and psychomotor scores. They found that those infants born to mothers with vitamin D deficiency scored lower in both mental and psychomotor tests than did the infants born to mothers who had higher vitamin D levels during pregnancy. The results showed a direct relationship between the mother's vitamin D level measured during pregnancy and both the mental and the psychomotor development of their offspring. That is, the higher the mother's pregnancy levels of vitamin D, the higher the mental and psychomotor development scores. Psychomotor scoring measures physical skills such as movement, coordination, and dexterity.

Also published in *Pediatrics* in 2012 was an Australian study that demonstrated significant language impairment at five and ten years of age in the offspring of mothers who had vitamin D deficiency during pregnancy. The researchers concluded that dietary supplementation with vitamin D in mothers during pregnancy may reduce the risk of developmental language difficulties among their children. In October 2012, yet another Australian study on vitamin D in pregnancy was published in *Pediatrics* journal. This one found that low levels of vitamin D in pregnancy could increase the likelihood of eczema in the first year of a child's life.

Further, in December 2012, the *Journal of Clinical Endocrinology & Metabolism* published results from a multicentre study that indicated that women deficient in vitamin D in the first three months of pregnancy are twice as likely to give birth to babies with lower birth weights ("small for gestational age"), suggesting growth restriction later in the pregnancy.

In the March 2013 issue of *The Journal of Allergy and Clinical Immunology* was an Australian study that found that one-year-old infants with vitamin D deficiency (less than 50 nmol/L) were more likely to be peanut and/or egg allergic than those infants with adequate vitamin D levels. The researchers concluded that vitamin D sufficiency may be an important protective factor for food allergy in the first year of life. This again reinforces the need for mothers to maintain a good level of vitamin D throughout pregnancy and while breast-feeding.

In April 2013, the journal *Cancer Epidemiology, Biomarkers, & Prevention* published the results of a large population-based case-control study in California, USA. It suggests that greater exposure to UV radiation (from sunlight) during pregnancy may decrease the odds of developing some childhood cancers such as acute lymphoblastic leukaemia, hepatoblastoma, and non-Hodgkin's lymphoma. This points to further studies to be conducted to understand better the role of vitamin D levels in such results.

In June 2013, an Australian study published in the *International Journal of Eating Disorders* showed the outcome of low vitamin D levels at midpregnancy in the frequency of eating disorders among teenage girls. The 526 participants in this study had their blood vitamin D levels measured at eighteen weeks of pregnancy. Their daughters were assessed for eating disorders at the ages of fourteen, seventeen, and twenty years. The researchers found that a significant prediction of eating disorders among these girls, relative to their mothers' vitamin D levels in mid-pregnancy. In those mothers falling within the lowest quarter of vitamin D blood-level results, their daughters were more than twice as likely to have eating disorders than the daughters of mothers whose vitamin D levels fell within the top one-quarter of mid-pregnancy results.

There may be a longer-term effect on children relative to the vitamin D levels of their mothers during pregnancy. In January 2014, the *Journal of Clinical Endocrinology and Metabolism* published research showing that children are likely to have stronger muscles if their mothers have a higher level of vitamin D in their bodies during pregnancy. The University of Southampton researchers measured vitamin D levels in 678 women taking part in the Southampton Women's Survey, considered to be one of the largest and best characterized such studies globally. When their children were four years old, their grip strength and muscle mass were measured. Grip strength of the child was higher if his or her mother had higher body levels of vitamin D during pregnancy. There was also an association between the mother's vitamin D level and the child's muscle mass. The researchers concluded,

"These associations between maternal vitamin D and offspring muscle strength may well have consequences for later health."

In these more recent studies, we see a greater emphasis for pregnant women to consult with their doctors on blood tests for vitamin D status and to take remedial action if those levels of this important vitamin are low. A position statement of the Australian and New Zealand Bone and Mineral Society and Osteoporosis Australia recently provided guidelines for pregnant women, which include a recommendation that pregnant women should be screened routinely for vitamin D deficiency at their first prenatal visit. Even though women found to have vitamin D deficiency were prescribed vitamin D supplements, those women also should be screened again at twenty-eight weeks of pregnancy.

Adequacy of vitamin D is determined via a blood test showing a level of 25(OH)D, which is greater than 50 nmol/L. Those pregnant women tested at their first antenatal visit who have levels lower than this would be advised to take one capsule of vitamin D (1000 IU) daily. (Note that 1,000 IU = 25 µg [25 micrograms] of vitamin D). Those whose test shows 25(OH)D levels lower than 30 nmol/L would be advised to start with two capsules of vitamin D 1000 IU daily (that is, 2000 IU or 50 µg per day). Vitamin D supplementation should be considered throughout both pregnancy and breast-feeding.

One source of vitamin D is, surprisingly, fish. Although fish cannot synthesize vitamin D or provitamin D, both originate at the beginning of the food chain in phytoplankton.

THE NEED FOR FOLATE

Like vitamin D, adequacy of folate is important, both before conception and throughout the pregnancy. In "*Expecting the 'Expecting,'*" I mentioned the need for a woman to be on folate supplements at least one month, and preferably three months, before conception to avoid the debilitating condition of spina bifida in newborns. That is the ideal situation if a choice is made to initiate a pregnancy and if planning takes place well in advance of becoming pregnant.

Life does not always provide us with such early decisions; pregnancy can occur rather unexpectedly. It is for this reason that many countries either have, or will soon have, legislation dictating the folate enrichment of items such as bread so that the majority of women of childbearing age will already have adequate folate in their bodies at the time of conception. Food fortification with folic acid is already mandatory in seventy-five nations, and it is reported that requirement has resulted in a 50 to 70 percent reduction in neural-tube defects in those areas. However, governments in Europe and in many parts of Asia have so far neglected mandatory fortification.

Spina bifida is particularly debilitating for babies and children. The name of the condition is Latin for "split spine." It describes a developmental problem very early in the fœtus when some of the vertebrae intended to cover and protect the spinal cord do not form fully, and some spinal cord nerves do not develop normally. As a result, nerves are exposed or unprotected and may protrude through the gap in the vertebrae. A wide range of organs, muscles, and bodily functions that are dependent on nerves below the gap in the incomplete vertebrae are usually affected. Although the "split spine" can be closed surgically following birth, this does not restore normal function to those areas of the spinal cord that have become affected.

The risk of spina bifida is approximately one in every one thousand pregnancies. However, if the mother takes folate supplements beginning at least one month (preferably three months) before conception and continuing daily throughout the first three months of pregnancy, it can reduce the risk of spina bifida by up to 70 percent.

A Norwegian study published in the *Journal of the American Medical Association* (*JAMA*) in 2013 studied development outcomes in 85,176 children and concluded that the *"use or prenatal folic acid supplements around the time of conception was associated with a lower risk of autistic disorder in this group of children."* The researchers believed that this study supported prenatal folic acid supplementation. The children of those mothers who had taken folic acid supplements from four weeks before to eight weeks after the start of their pregnancies had an incidence of autism only less than one-half that of the children whose mothers had not taken folic acid supplements for that period.

This study reinforces the need for folate supplements. An earlier Norwegian study found that maternal folic acid supplementation taken from four weeks before to eight weeks after conception was associated with a reduced risk of severe language delay in three-year-old children.

An Australian study published in the *Journal of the American Association for Cancer Research* in 2012 concluded that this study provided evidence for a specific protective effect of prenatal folic acid supplements against the risk of childhood brain tumours when the supplements are taken before and possibly during pregnancy.

The recommended level of folate supplementation is at least 400 µg/d (400 micrograms per day of folic acid), but unless a woman is consuming ample amounts of folate-enriched breakfast cereals, breads, and food beverages, then consuming tablets containing 500 µg or 800 µg of folic acid daily would be preferable. Foods naturally high in folate include green leafy vegetables (e.g., broccoli, spinach, and salad greens); chickpeas; nuts; and orange juice. Pregnancy involves a greater requirement for folic acid and, for the benefits outlined above, folate supplementation should be continued throughout pregnancy.

SELENIUM – A "NUTTY" SOLUTION

The trace mineral selenium is an essential nutrient of fundamental importance to human health. Selenium is the basis for important antioxidant enzymes because it is incorporated into proteins to make selenoproteins. Through their antioxidant properties, selenoproteins help prevent the cell-damaging effects of free radicals. Other selenoproteins play a role in the immune system.

Selenium enters the food chain through plants, which take the element up from the soil. Plants grown in regions where the soil is low in selenium do not provide meaningful amounts of selenium to people who eat them. Although selenium can be found in some meats, animals that are raised in regions with low selenium levels will accumulate low levels of selenium within their muscle tissues.

Regions with low soil levels of selenium include Denmark, Finland, eastern and central Siberia (Russia), an area extending from northeast to south-central China, Western Australia, and New Zealand. Although there appear to be other areas with low soil selenium, they have not been subject to intensive research.

Dairy products and eggs contribute small amounts of selenium to the diet. There is a dominance of cereal-based foods as core sources of selenium — if those cereals are sourced from regions with good soil levels of selenium. An interesting example is that wheat grown in the eastern states of Australia and imported into New Zealand has resulted in significant improvement in the normally low selenium levels within the New Zealand population.

The low blood selenium concentrations in New Zealanders have prompted much research on selenium in recent decades. A study by the Department of Nutrition, University of Otago, Dunedin, New Zealand, and published in *The American Journal of Clinical Nutrition* in 2008, found that the consumption of just two Brazil nuts per day is an effective way of increasing selenium status. The researchers concluded, "Inclusion of this high-selenium food in the diet could avoid the need for fortification (of other foods) or supplements to improve the selenium status of New Zealanders."

Ocean fish are also a moderately good source of selenium, although they provide considerably less selenium than Brazil nuts. If you decide to obtain your selenium from Brazil nuts, then you do not need to take supplementary selenium products. Eating Brazil nuts *and* taking selenium supplementary products may cause you to exceed the recommended upper limits for selenium intake (400 micrograms per day). There is an interrelationship between iodine and selenium; therefore, it is recommended that you accompany selenium supplementation with simultaneous iodine supplementation (see the next chapter).

Because many regions of the world have selenium-deficient soils, you may be wise to *either* take selenium supplements (200 micrograms per day) *or* eat two Brazil nuts per day.

The interaction between selenium and iodine remains unclear. It is felt that if iodine levels are very low, then selenium supplementation may worsen iodine deficiency. For this reason, selenium supplementation also should be accompanied by simultaneous iodine supplementation.

IODINE

Soils in various regions around the world also can be deficient in iodine, often in the same regions where soils are very low in selenium — for example, in New Zealand and in parts of Australia, such as Tasmania. Many decades ago, the frequency of *iodine-deficiency goitre* (enlargement of the thyroid gland, situated at the base of the throat), resulted in some authorities taking action to encourage the use of commercially manufactured household salt fortified with iodine. This action was successful in avoiding development of goitre within those populations.

In more recent decades, three situations have taken place that have resulted in the loss of this protection:

1. Domestically, both for cooking and for table salt, households moved from commercially manufactured salt to raw "rock salt," which has lower or absent iodine content.

2. There has been a move to more frequent restaurant dining and/or consumption of "fast foods," following the major increase in retail outlets providing these heavily advertised

foods. These food sources use bulk raw-salt supplies rather than commercially manufactured, iodine-fortified salt.

3. Concerns about possible adverse health effects from the excessive intake of salt have prompted households to reduce their use of added salt during meals.

As a result, iodine deficiency again has become evident within these populations, with enlarged thyroid glands indicating an increased risk of developing goitre.

We have known for quite some time that severe iodine deficiency during pregnancy can have a direct adverse effect on fœtal brain development, which is associated with a subsequent and significant negative effect on babies' mental development. Not so broadly acknowledged has been the long-term impact on children of even mild iodine deficiency during their mothers' pregnancies.

In April 2013, *The Journal of Clinical Endocrinology & Metabolism* published the outcome of an Australian study on nine-year-old children born to mothers with differing iodine levels during pregnancy. Those children whose mothers had mild iodine deficiency during pregnancy had reductions of 10 percent in spelling, 7.6 percent in grammar, and 5.7 percent in English literacy, compared with children whose mothers had appropriate levels of iodine during pregnancy. The researchers concluded that even mild iodine deficiency during pregnancy can adversely impact fœtal neurodevelopment that does not appear to be compensated by providing iodine sufficiency during childhood.

In May 2013, *The Lancet* medical journal published a study conducted in England looking at the effect of inadequate iodine status during pregnancy on cognitive outcomes in children. The children from single births in 1,040 women had IQ testing at eight years of age and were assessed for reading ability at nine years of age. More than two-thirds of the women in this study were found to have mild to moderate iodine deficiency, and their offspring were much more likely to have test scores that fell within the lowest quarter in verbal IQ, reading comprehension, and reading accuracy, The researchers concluded that these results emphasize the importance of adequate iodine status early in pregnancy, particularly with regard to the long-term risk iodine deficiency can pose to a developing infant. They believe that iodine deficiency in pregnant women should be regarded as an important public health issue that needs attention.

The consumption of rich sources of iodine such as eggs, ocean fish, and dairy products can help reduce the likelihood of iodine deficiency. But because adequate iodine is important as early as in the first trimester (first three months) of pregnancy, it is prudent to take iodine supplements as soon as pregnancy is confirmed. After earlier studies in Australia showed that mild iodine deficiency was rather general, since 2009, iodized salt has replaced noniodized salt in all bread sold in Australia.

The Dietary Reference Intake (Food and Nutrition Board, Institute of Medicine, USA) provides a Recommended Dietary Allowance (RDA) for iodine for nonpregnant women and also for men of 150 µg (150 micrograms, or mcg) per day. For pregnant women, the recommendation is an RDA of 220 µg per day. Women who normally consume food items regarded as rich in iodine do not need to take an additional 220 µg per day of iodine supplementation. This is why dietary supplements specifically intended for pregnancy contain lesser amounts as in, for example, Blackmores "I-Folic™," which provides 150 µg iodine plus 500 µg folic acid.

As explained at the end of the previous chapter, if supplementation of selenium is required, then simultaneous iodine supplementation also should be taken.

ZINC

More than 200 *metallo-enzymes* within our bodies incorporate zinc. A metallo-enzyme is an enzyme that incorporates a metallic ion. Those metallo-enzymes that contain zinc have numerous important functions within the body. Therefore, where there is zinc deficiency, immune function can be compromised, stunted growth can occur, brain and eye function can be affected, and behavioural disturbances may become apparent. In the brain, zinc-containing neurons appear to be associated with episodic memory function and are important for behaviour, emotional expression, and cognitive operations. Poor pregnancy outcome has been noted in cases of zinc deficiency. In babies, low maternal zinc intake has been associated with lessened attention during the neonatal period and worse motor functioning at six months of age.

If a healthy, well-balanced daily diet is consumed, then zinc deficiency is not common. Red meat provides a good source of zinc, as does seafood — oysters are one of the richest sources of dietary zinc. Nuts and milk are also good sources of zinc.

During pregnancy, there are high fœtal requirements for zinc, so those women who start their pregnancies with a marginal zinc status have an increased risk of becoming zinc-deficient.

The bioavailability to the body of zinc consumed from vegetarian diets is lower than that from nonvegetarian diets. Meat is high in bioavailable zinc, and the meat protein may enhance zinc absorption. However, vegetarians typically eat high levels of legumes and whole grains, which contain phytates that tend to bind zinc and inhibit its absorption. For this reason, vegetarians often require as much as 50 percent more zinc supplementation than nonvegetarians.

During periods of rapid growth, such as pregnancy and infancy, is when people are most susceptible to zinc deficiency. Animal studies have shown that zinc deprivation during early development causes irreversible impairment of normal brain development. If zinc supplements are taken, then the daily zinc intake from supplements should not exceed 25 mg per day. Studies on zinc supplementation in pregnant women with low levels of zinc during early pregnancy have shown significantly higher birth weight and larger infant head circumference relative to similar women who were not supplemented with zinc. This result was achieved on a daily supplementary dose of 25 mg of zinc per day.

HELPING BABY'S BRAIN DEVELOPMENT

Possibly the most significant discovery in infant development since science-based attention turned to seeking what may influence brain development, cognition, and intelligence was an appreciation that nutrition can play an important role. At one time, it was considered that the key to higher intelligence was a matter of "selecting your own parents." Genetics probably do have a positive influence. Then a key factor was considered to be "the environment." It is now apparent that families in which parents allocate a lot of "quality time" to their babies and children usually have brighter children. That is not too surprising given that babies are like little "sponges," absorbing far more from their surroundings than we give them credit for, with an inherent ability to learn at surprising rates. The brain has a tendency to develop better when it is "challenged." However, over the past few decades, and especially within the past twenty years, a greater appreciation has taken place of the role of nutrition both in the womb and during the first two years of life in enhancing brain development.

The first nutrient that linked deficiency during pregnancy and early childhood with long-term adverse effects on scholastic achievement and behaviour was iron. In 1985, adequate iron intake (as outlined in "*The Importance of Iron*") was shown to be critical.

In the second half of pregnancy, the brain of the developing baby grows at a rate that can be described as nothing short of phenomenal. By the end of the second trimester (twenty-seven weeks), the average brain weight of the fœtus is about 115 g. At full term (forty weeks), the average brain weighs about 360 g. That is threefold increase in brain weight during the third trimester.

Neurons are already beginning to be formed as early as the seventh week of pregnancy, but the great majority of neurons are generated during the second trimester. The development of each neuron involves three primary steps:

1. *Proliferation*, when the neurons are generated within the central area of the brain

2. *Migration*, as the newly generated neurons move from the proliferative zone toward the positions they will assume in the developing cortex of the brain

3. *Differentiation*, when the neurons reach their destination in the neocortex and develop the structural and molecular elements that will allow them to connect with other neurons to exert their functional roles

It is estimated that by full-term birth, approximately one hundred billion neurons make up the central nervous system (CNS). That is 100,000,000,000 neurons! It has been estimated that during the peak period of proliferation, in excess of two hundred thousand neurons are being generated *every minute*! However, by the last weeks of the second trimester, neuron production is essentially complete, and the generation of the supporting glial cells is in progress.

What does this tell us? It should tell us that throughout pregnancy, consideration for your rapidly developing baby dictates healthy eating that can support his or her growth and mental development requirements at all times. It should also tell us that the rapidly developing brain should be protected from harmful substances such as maternal intake of alcohol, recreational drugs, drugs of dependency, and the toxic by-products of inhaled cigarette smoke.

When we consider the extremely high rate of cell division taking place *every second* and *every minute* as your baby's brain develops, then *"just a glass or two of alcohol should be OK"* or *"just one more cigarette will not hurt"* is unacceptable. Ingesting these substances places at risk all of those thousands of important cells that are actively dividing and developing in your baby's brain at that particular time. Also, because recreational drugs affect an adult's brain processes, then we should stop and think what brain pathways will be affected in the very rapidly developing brain of a fœtus during that period while his or her mother has a recreational drug in her system.

As I mentioned in my first chapter, there are multiple levels of timing, and each plays an important role in shaping the developing brain. Once the time for a particular phase of brain growth has passed, it cannot be restarted.

A healthy diet is not the only factor that can influence the development of your baby's brain. Healthy exercise also may play an important role. In more recent times, science has helped us understand that, in adulthood, regular exercise improves blood flow to the brain. For many people, as we get older, exercise can slow the progression of age-related dementia and Alzheimer's disease. New studies are suggesting that regular healthy exercise during pregnancy may boost the baby's brain development. Montreal researchers reported to the Neuroscience 2013 Congress held in San Diego, California, USA, their finding that even twenty minutes of moderate exercise three times each week during pregnancy gave infants a head start — and that this benefit could continue on much later in life. Their study, the first random-controlled trial in humans, reinforced similar results in earlier animal studies.

When we were conceived, our mothers most probably were advised to "take it easy" during pregnancy. It is now considered that such inactivity might have been more harmful to both mother and baby than exercise and that, instead, moderate healthy exercise during pregnancy not only benefits the mother but also provides her baby with a better start to brain development that may persist for many years ahead.

Research over the past two decades has progressively established the major influence that a good dietary intake of *"essential"* fatty acids, both during pregnancy and in the feeding of babies after they are born, can have on brain development into childhood. Of particular interest is the Omega-3 long-chain polyunsaturated fatty acid (LCPUFA) docosahexaenoic acid (DHA).

THOSE "ESSENTIAL" OMEGA-3 FATTY ACIDS

"Fatty" acids are the individual molecules that make up the general fats in our diet or serve many important functions in our bodies. Many of these fatty acids can be manufactured from scratch by metabolic processes within our bodies, then further modified to larger fatty acid molecules. Specific enzyme systems within our bodies assist in these modifications. Some larger fatty acid molecules are extremely important to our health and well-being, yet our bodies lack the enzyme systems to form them. These fatty acids instead must be taken in as part of our diet; therefore, they are known as *"essential fatty acids"* — that is, it is *essential* that they are present within our diet because our bodies are simply unable to form them.

Although they share the same metabolic enzyme systems, these essential fatty acids are categorized into two groups: the "Omega-6 fatty acids" and the "Omega-3 fatty acids," according to their molecular structure. Both groups are polyunsaturated fatty acids (PUFAs). Those that are present in plant sources (e.g., in vegetable oils) are the Omega-6 linoleic acid (LA) and the

Omega-3 alpha-linolenic acid (aLA). In theory, the enzyme systems in our bodies are able to metabolize these PUFAs through the addition of more carbon atoms and greater "desaturation" to form larger molecules known as "long-chain polyunsaturated fatty acids" (LCPUFAs). The body's ability to have them undergo this metabolism is very restricted; therefore, these LCPUFAs must be present in our diet from sources where they have already been formed.

The key Omega-6 LCPUFA is arachidonic acid (ARA). The key Omega-3 LCPUFAs are eicosapentaenoic acid (EPA) and docosahexaenoic acid (DHA).

By the time a baby is born, its brain weighs about 360 g (13 oz.). Rapid brain growth during the first twelve months of life increases brain weight to approximately 1,000 g (2 lb., 3 oz.). A slower rate of growth in the next twelve months increases the weight of the brain to approximately 1,200 g at two years of age. Not much increase in the weight of the brain occurs after that; the average adult male brain weighs approximately 1,400 g (3 lb., 1 oz.) and the average adult female brain weighs approximately 1,250 g (2 lb., 12 oz.). My wife explains to me that women use their brains more efficiently!

From the end of the second trimester (at about six months of pregnancy), the developing baby's brain begins to incorporate increasing amounts of Omega-3 DHA and Omega-6 ARA LCPUFAs.

This rapid uptake of these two essential fatty acids continues until two years of age before slowing in the third year of life.

The brain does not take in the PUFAs linoleic acid and alpha-linolenic acid.

During pregnancy, the fœtus takes from its mother as much DHA as possible by a selective process of the placenta known as "*bio-magnification*", resulting in a far greater concentration of DHA in the fœtal circulation than in the maternal circulation. This preferential placental transfer of DHA to the fœtus takes place at the "expense" of the mother's DHA status. Such a mechanism helps protect the supply of DHA to the fœtus during a critical period of development. Of course, sufficiency for the developing baby can take place only if the mother has an adequate intake of DHA from her diet.

What happens if the fœtus does not get from its mother enough DHA to meet its requirements for optimum brain development, visual development, and general cell membrane building, processes that need DHA? Would this mean that new cells are not formed, or the fœtus dies? No. The body then uses "the next best thing" for these cell structures in place of unavailable DHA. The "substitute" fatty acid for DHA in the brain and the retina of the eye is usually the Omega-6 docosapentaenoic acid (DPA). This is not an Omega-3 fatty acid like DHA and EPA. While the recipient cell can still function with the substituted Omega-6 DPA, it is unlikely to be able to do so with the same efficiency and efficacy as it would have been able to achieve with Omega-3 DHA. Omega-3 LCPUFA deficiency is usually associated with visual and cognitive deficits.

A Norwegian study published in the prestigious medical journal *Pediatrics* in 2003 clearly showed that a good maternal intake of Omega-3 LCPUFA during pregnancy and breast-feeding had a favourable effect on later mental development in children. In this study, participating women were assigned randomly to either of two regimens to be taken daily from eighteen weeks of pregnancy until three months of breast-feeding:

1. Capsules of 10 ml of cod liver oil containing:
   a. 1,183 mg Omega-3 docosahexaenoic acid (DHA)
   b. 803 mg Omega-3 eicosapentaenoic acid (EPA)

2. Capsules of 10 ml of corn oil containing:
   a. 4,747 mg Omega-6 linoleic acid (LA)
   b. 92 mg Omega-3 alpha-linolenic acid (aLA)

The amount of the fat-soluble vitamins A, D, and E were identical in the two oils.

From three months of age, the babies from both groups received daily cod liver oil in line with Norwegian-recommended guidelines for infant nutrition.

Intelligence testing using the K-ABC was conducted with children from both groups at four years of age. The Kaufman Assessment Battery for Children (K-ABC) is commonly used, mainly in Europe, as a measure of intelligence and achievement designed for children aged 2.5 years through 12.5 years. The children in both groups were assessed on sequential processing, simultaneous processing, and nonverbal abilities. Scores from sequential processing and simultaneous processing are combined to form a Mental Processing Composite that serves as the measure of intelligence in the K-ABC.

Children who were born to mothers in the cod liver oil (high Omega-3 LCPUFA intake) group scored significantly higher on the Mental Processing Composite of the K-ABC at four years of age than the children whose mothers were in the corn-oil group. The researchers in this study found that the children's mental development scores at four years of age correlated significantly with maternal intake of DHA and EPA during pregnancy.

Of interest in this study is that the "base" DHA status of these women who were Scandinavian (and therefore probably had a relatively high fish intake) already would have been good — as evidenced by the breast-milk DHA level of 0.47 percent of total fatty acids in the "placebo" (corn-oil capsules) group at three months of breast-feeding. This DHA level would be higher than that in the breast milk of mothers in most other populations.

A key takeaway from this study is that even if a mother already has a good DHA status, supplementary DHA taken during pregnancy can provide further long-lasting benefit for her infant. For mothers with a "poor" DHA status, supplementary DHA during pregnancy is even more important.

A suitable supplementary intake of Omega-3 DHA during pregnancy (and during breast-feeding) would be in the order of 1,000 mg per day, which is close to that consumed by the mothers taking 10 ml of cod liver oil in the study mentioned above. Do not confuse "1,000 mg" of DHA with fish-oil capsules in the marketplace labelled "Fish Oil 1,000" capsules. In these, "1,000" refers to the total fish-oil content (1,000 mg) of each capsule. However, the DHA content of each capsule is usually just 120 mg per capsule, requiring that you take about eight capsules per day! Because each "Fish Oil 1000" capsule usually also contains 180 mg of another important Omega-3, EPA, an intake of eight capsules per day would provide almost 1,500 mg of EPA, which is more than is probably required. The study mentioned above provided only about one-half of that amount of EPA to the mothers who were taking the cod liver oil.

I would recommend an amount similar to that which I take daily for my own general well-being. In Australia, a Blackmores product branded "Omega Brain" contains in each capsule 500 mg of DHA and 100 mg EPA. By taking just one of these capsules each day together with just three capsules of Fish Oil 1000, I have a daily supplementary intake as follows:

Capsules	Total DHA	Total EPA
1 x Omega Brain	500 mg	100 mg
3 x Fish Oil 1000	360 mg	540 mg
Total Omega-3	860 mg	640 mg

This supplementary intake of important Omega-3 together with inclusion of suitable fish in the diet will provide a good total intake of both DHA and EPA during pregnancy. This amount will help ensure a good start to life for your new baby and will provide ample DHA for good brain development during the period of development in the womb and early infancy, resulting in long-term benefits.

The findings in this Norwegian study are well supported by the benefits to brain and eye development that result from an adequate provision of DHA to babies during babyhood. This has been shown clinically in several studies, whether the babies received the adequate amounts of DHA from breast milk or from one of the few baby formulas that contains a level of DHA that equals the average level of DHA found in sixty-seven breast-milk studies from around the world. Such a baby formula contains 17 mg of DHA per 100 kcal (418 kj).

In 1986, published research provided evidence that Omega-3 fatty acids were essential for brain and eye development. In the United States, President George H. W. Bush designated the 1990s as "The Decade of the Brain," and substantial government funding was made available to researchers. The aim may have been to understand the human brain better as a means to improve computers, but the research performed was valuable in understanding the benefits to babies that accrue from them receiving an adequate intake of LCPUFA essential fatty acids.

In the year 2000, clinical studies began to be published in key, peer-reviewed medical journals revealing the significant benefits in mental development index (MDI) scores in babies who were fed baby formula that contained adequate amounts of the LCPUFAs Omega-3 DHA and Omega-6 ARA. MDI scoring is similar to IQ scoring, and the average score is 100. Babies who had been fed formula with LCPUFA during their first seventeen weeks achieved, on average at eighteen months of age, an MDI score seven points higher than babies fed the same formula without the LCPUFA content (the "control" formula). The fact that 26 percent of these babies scored 115 (seventeen points higher than the average for the babies on the control formula) prompted *Scientific American* magazine to take the unprecedented step of highlighting the study as a "Formula for Intelligence?" The researchers commented, "These data support a long-term cognitive advantage of infant DHA supply during the first four months of life."

High intelligence scores were not the only benefit gained by babies who received adequate amounts of DHA. Studies published that same year showed that babies who were fed formula containing LCPUFA had significantly better visual function at twelve months of age than babies on the control formula (without DHA). The following year (2001), the *Journal of Pediatrics* published a clinical study that found a significant connection between DHA in a baby's diet and language performance at nine months of age.

Grants from the National Institutes of Health in the United States supported these studies, and further studies conducted at the Retina Foundation of the Southwest in Dallas, Texas, confirmed greater visual and neural development in babies who were fed formula that contained DHA. The longer a period of time that babies were fed formula with adequate levels of DHA (up to twelve months of age), the more their visual skills developed.[1]

A further endorsement for the benefits of babies receiving adequate amounts of LCPUFAs during rapid brain development comes from a study published in *The American Journal of Clinical Nutrition* in mid-2013. In this study, babies who had received baby formula containing adequate amounts throughout their first twelve months were tested every six months, from eighteen months of age to six years of age (seventy-two months of age). The tasks

---

1. More detailed information from these studies can be found in the book *How to Choose a Baby Formula*, also by Garry Wainscott, Amazon/Kindle, 2012.

administered during the preschool years focused on working memory, inhibitory control, attention flexibility, planning and strategy on various complex tasks, verbal performance, and intelligence. The various tests chosen were appropriate for age at each six-month testing. The study found that baby formula with adequate levels of LCPUFAs during the first twelve months of life had significant longer-term benefits into early childhood (from three to six years of life) in such areas as rule learning and inhibition tasks, vocabulary, and IQ compared to those children who had received baby formula without added LCPUFAs.

Also published in mid-2013 was a study conducted in Oxfordshire, UK, of 493 healthy schoolchildren aged seven to nine years who had below-average reading-performance assessments at age seven. It was found that their levels of the Omega-3 LCPUFAs — DHA and EPA — were low, and lower levels were directly related to measures of cognition and behaviour. Lower levels of DHA were associated with poorer reading ability.

From this extensive research base with consistent beneficial results for improvement in the early eye and brain development of babies and children, from their receipt of adequate long-chain Omega-3 DHA, both in the womb and following birth, it can be well appreciated just how important it is for mothers to take in their diets ample amounts of fish and DHA supplements throughout pregnancy.

THERE IS "OMEGA-3".... AND THEN THERE IS "OMEGA-3"

There is a lot of confusion among the general public, and even among some doctors, regarding what is referred to as "Omega-3" fatty acids. This confusion is the result of insufficient differentiation between Omega-3 polyunsaturated fatty acid (PUFA) and Omega-3 long-chain polyunsaturated fatty acids (LCPUFAs).

Omega-3 PUFA comes from plant-based sources such as flaxseed oil and soy oil. Omega-3 LCPUFAs come from animal-based sources such as fish oil and krill, and also from algae. Algal-based sources provide Omega-3 LCPUFA in a form that is suitable for vegetarians.

The human body can metabolize Omega-3 plant-based al-pha-linolenic acid PUFA to Omega-3 LCPUFAs. Unfortunately, however, studies over the past two decades clearly have shown that such conversion is of a very low order indeed. Provide in a breast-feeding mother's diet some oily fish, and her breast milk DHA level is elevated. Provide in her diet flaxseed oil, and there is no increase whatsoever in her breast-milk DHA. Sophisticated scientific studies indicate that when plant-based Omega-3 PUFA is taken in the diet, a large amount of it is used quickly as a source of energy for the body.

Researchers generally agree that whole-body conversion of alpha-linolenic acid (Omega-3 PUFA) to DHA is below 5 percent in humans. The metabolism of both Omega-3 fatty acids and Omega-6 fatty acids in the body share, and compete for, the same enzymes. Thus, the efficiency of Omega-3 metabolism can be affected adversely by a high concentration of Omega-6 fatty acids and Omega-6 LCPUFAs in the diet. High amounts of Omega-6 fatty acids (for example, linoleic acid, which is prevalent in most vegetable oils) in the diet tend to reduce further the conversion rate of Omega-3 PUFA to Omega-3 LCPUFAs.

Not only the amount but also the "balance" between Omega-6 LCPUFAs and Omega-3 LCPUFAs in the diet can affect immune function. Many studies have been published over the past decade showing not only this effect but also a possible impact on the greatly increased incidence in baby and child allergies we have been witnessing in recent years.

Some will attribute that to "the hygiene factor," whose logic is that, in recent years, we have tried hard to keep our children as "clean" as possible. In so doing, we have prevented their exposure to the general environment within which children can naturally develop immunities to what surrounds them.

However, growing evidence shows that high dietary intake of Omega-6 LCPUFAs tends to have a "pro-inflammatory" effect, whereas Omega-3 LCPUFAs tend to have an "anti-inflammatory" effect, helping keep inflammation under control. Modern Western diets have resulted in the composition of breast-milk fatty acids changing significantly over the past twenty years or so, reflecting the increase in dietary Omega-6 LCPUFAs at the same time that the consumption of Omega-3 LCPUFAs has decreased.

It is now more widely accepted that, rather than high blood cholesterol levels themselves causing our cardiac problems, it is more an issue of inflammatory processes, some of which might be triggered by such things as viral infections, which, in turn, use cholesterol as a salve or "bandage" in inflamed blood vessels. Our dietary changes over recent decades may have played a hand in that.

This dietary evolution is not surprising. Some twenty-five to thirty years ago, there was a growing belief that our intake of saturated fats, particularly those in dairy products such as butter and full-fat milk, was killing us off with heart arrests from cardiac blood-vessel cholesterol plaque. This prompted a big shift from cooking with animal fats to the use of vegetable oils, mostly seed oils. The outcome was a significant increase in the consumption of Omega-6 fatty acids.

Soon thereafter, the alarmists had us avoiding or minimizing fish intake so that we were not exposed to methyl mercury. The result was a marked reduction in dietary Omega-3 LCPUFA fatty acids. And the now-ubiquitous availability of "fast foods" has helped exacerbate this major dietary shift. Whether or not this major change in dietary habits was justified has come into question more recently. Some saturated fats have become more "acceptable" as we are encouraged to turn back to consuming dairy products. Eggs are no longer blacklisted because their meagre contribution to cholesterol (remembering that most of our cholesterol is generated within the body, rather than from diet) is more than offset by the other valuable nutrients that eggs provide. The realization that the mercury content in marine foods is high mainly in those species at the end of the food chain such as shark and marlin allows us to return to eating other "healthy" species of fish.

We are currently faced with the fact that in many populations, our intake of Omega-6 fatty acids remains too high, and our intake of Omega-3 LCPUFAs is too low. The ratio of Omega-6 to Omega-3 in our daily diet should be about 2.3 to 1. However, studies in the United States have shown that over the past many decades, there has been a major shift of this ratio to a present-day ratio of about 10 to 1 or 15 to 1. Some ratios in the United States have even gone to 30 to 1. Acknowledging that Omega-6 fatty acids are regarded as "pro-inflammatory" and Omega-3 LCPUFAs are "anti-inflammatory," these changes in ratio can have significant impact on chronic disease states.

Of all types of food intake, the type of fats that are taken in from the diet can have an immediate impact on body fatty acids. In the case of fats, literally "we are what we eat," and it is virtually reflected on a day-to-day basis. Whether we are looking at what we are passing on to the fœtus in the womb, or to the baby being breast-fed, what you are eating is what your baby in the womb or your baby on the breast is also receiving.

Taking this into consideration, the type of fat taken in from your diet during pregnancy and/or during breast-feeding can have a profound effect on your baby now and for quite some time into his or her future. This is not only relative to brain and eye development but also to immunity and allergy. This should be an awakening for those who have long promoted that "breast is best" — are they talking about the breast milk of decades ago, with low Omega-6 and high Omega-3, or "present-day" breast milk, with its extremely high Omega-6 and rather low Omega-3?

A high ratio of Omega-6 to Omega-3 dietary intake may have other implications beyond immunity and allergy. In a study published in the *Journal of Clinical Endocrinology and Metabolism* in

January 2013, it was found that the children of mothers with a high level of Omega-6 PUFA during pregnancy showed an increased tendency toward higher body fat, but not to greater height. The higher the mother's plasma Omega-6 level when measured at thirty-four weeks of pregnancy, the greater was the tendency to obesity in their children when measured at four years and again at six years of life. This study concluded that a low intake of Omega-6 fatty acids by mothers during pregnancy might reduce the amount of adiposity (obesity) in their offspring.

During pregnancy and breast-feeding, there is a need to reduce the intake of seed vegetable oils with high Omega-6 content, such as soy oil, sunflower oil, corn oil, and safflower oil. Olive oil, with its high mono-unsaturated Omega-9 fatty-acid content, is a healthy vegetable oil, as is canola oil. Equally important is an effort to consume within the diet the "anti-inflammatory" Omega-3 LCPUFAs, These dietary disciplines are likely to reduce the likelihood of inflammatory and immunological episodes.

This same dietary "rebalancing" has the significant advantage of providing your baby, both within the womb and when born, with the levels of Omega-3 LCPUFA in both the retina (for improved visual acuity) and the brain (for intelligence) needed for proper development in the start to life.

IT'S A BIT "FISHY"

There is no doubt that marine fish provide us with a great protein source. This seafood is a "whole" lean protein food that also brings with it many important nutrients, including Omega-3 LCPUFAs, iron, iodine, selenium, zinc, and vitamins A and D.

Some caution needs to be applied to the type of fish selected for inclusion in the diet during pregnancy. For example, although "basa" (or "bassa"), the catfish from Vietnam, has a delightful texture that makes it pleasant to eat, it has a very low Omega-3 content—about one-quarter of the amount (by weight) of Omega-3 in Australian barramundi, snapper, trevally, dory, or hoki (blue grenadier). Rainbow trout provides twenty times more Omega-3 than basa, and Atlantic salmon provides thirty times more Omega-3 than basa.

Usually, cold-water deep-sea fish contain high levels of Omega-3 (the reason why my preferred dinner fish is New Zealand deep-sea dory), but a major exception is orange roughy; it contains negligible amounts of Omega-3. It depends to a large extent on what they eat in their natural environment. Shark (flake) also contains very little Omega-3 — only `about one-half that of basa. But you should avoid eating shark, so far up the food chain, for other reasons as well. (See the next chapter, "*Minimizing Mercury*").

Bream and silver perch are good sources of Omega-3, as are green-lipped mussels and oysters. If you are partial to smoked Atlantic salmon, then go for the "cold-smoked" salmon, which has a higher Omega-3 content than when it is "hot-smoked."

MINIMIZING MERCURY

Mercury is regarded as a global pollutant. While mercury occurs naturally within our environment, the period of significant industrial activity over the past two hundred years tended to concentrate mercury in many centres around our world. This environmental mercury is concentrated largely in its inorganic (chemical) form at first, but then by various methods it can become methyl mercury, which has high toxicity in humans. Microbes have the ability to synthesize inorganic mercury into methyl mercury. This methyl mercury can accumulate in various organisms, and as these organisms enter the basic food chain, methyl mercury can become concentrated in organisms farther up the food chain, a process known as *biomagnification.*

Sulphate- and iron-reducing bacteria have the ability to methylate mercury in low-oxygen environments, like, for example, in the beds of lakes, slow-flowing streams, and rivers; they enter the food chain from there. These organisms may be consumed by higher organisms, which may be consumed by small fish. These fish are consumed by larger predatory fish, which are, in turn, consumed by even larger fish, so biomagnification takes place. This suggests that eating larger fish such as sharks, which are at the top of the marine food chain on a frequent

77

basis, might mean that the intake of toxic methyl mercury would be undesirable. Even tuna tend to have significant mercury levels and therefore should not be consumed with great frequency.

Regions of past or recent heavy industrial concentration, such as in parts of Europe, the United States, or Japan, may have a legacy of significant mercury entry into the environment. In the United States, there are lakes, rivers, and streams where signs warn visitors that fish taken from these bodies of water should not be consumed. However, in other regions in our world, there is far less concern about methyl mercury pollution if local fish are being eaten. It's important to note that many species of shark that travel great distances might not be regarded as "local."

Several years ago, I was instrumental in setting up a multicentre breast-milk study among mothers in three regions of Sri Lanka — in a major fishing village; in the capital city of Colombo; and in Kandy, nestled in the central hills district. We were investigating the impact of maternal diet on breast-milk content of Omega-3 DHA. Not unexpectedly, we found that the breast milk of mothers around the fishing villages was double that of the mothers living in the central hills, well away from fresh fish sources.

I had the eight most commonly consumed fish in Sri Lanka analyzed, not only for Omega-3, but also for mercury. These analyses were carried out both by the Department of Nutrition at the University of Otago in Dunedin, New Zealand, and by the Government Science Laboratories in Perth, Western Australia. The analytical results were amazingly consistent between the two laboratories. The level of mercury in Sri Lankan fish was virtually nonexistent and inconsequential.

Before and during pregnancy, an effort should be made to minimize the intake of mercury from food, and it becomes very much a balancing act. On the one hand, mercury exposure from the consumption of some species of fish may give rise to accumulating body mercury in the mother, which she passes on to the developing fœtus. On the other hand, twice-weekly consumption of other species of fish during pregnancy appears to have a protective effect. For example, a recently published (October 2012) long-term study carried out in the United States and supported by grants from the National Institute of Environmental Health Sciences, National Institutes of Health, analyzed the outcome of mercury exposure (measured by mercury level in the hair of mothers soon after giving birth) on ADHD-related behaviour of their children, who were examined at eight years of age. Their results revealed the following:

- Mercury exposure in mothers is associated with ADHD in their children.

- The risk for these behaviours increased in line with the mother's hair mercury levels soon after birth.

- The children of mothers consuming at least two servings of fish per week during pregnancy had a decrease in ADHD behaviours, especially in impulsivity/hyperactivity.

It would appear, then, that the benefits of nutrients in fish for the brain of the developing fœtus may outweigh some of the deleterious effects of low-level mercury exposure.

However, be aware that the high mercury levels in some fish in some locales do pose a risk. Personally, I eat New Zealand deep-sea dory. It is caught in the near-pristine waters of the southern oceans toward Antarctica, it is not a predatory fish toward the top of the food chain, and it has a high DHA content.

LISTERIOSIS

Listeriosis is a serious infection usually caused by eating food that is contaminated with the bacterium *Listeria monocytogenes*. Pregnancy brings with it a higher risk of contracting an infection. Listeriosis is an important public-health problem that primarily affects older adults, pregnant women, newborn babies, and adults who have weakened immune systems. The risk may be reduced through safe food preparation, consumption, and storage.

Pregnant women are about thirteen to twenty times more likely than other healthy adults to contract listeriosis. Although the symptoms of listeriosis in pregnant women are usually only mild, or even absent, infections may result in miscarriage, premature labour, and serious illness or death in newborn babies. Babies born with *Listeria* infection may develop septicæmia or meningitis.

During pregnancy, if you develop fever or nonspecific symptoms such as fatigue and aches, it is advisable to consult with your doctor within twenty-four hours. If you have been infected, then appropriate antibiotics will protect your unborn or newborn baby.

To reduce the risk of contracting *Listeria*, it is best to avoid the following foods:

- Milk that has not been pasteurized. Do not drink raw (unpasteurized) milk; drink or use only milk that you are confident has been pasteurized. The American Academy of Pediatrics (AAP) recently called for a ban on the sale of unpasteurized milk and milk products throughout the United States because of the "significant health risk" to pregnant women, infants, and children. The US Food and Drug Administration currently prohibits the sale of unpasteurized milk across state borders in the United States, but the AAP is seeking a total ban nationwide because the consumption of raw milk and raw-milk products can result in severe and life-threatening illnesses such as miscarriage and stillbirths in pregnant women, as well as meningitis and blood-borne infections in both young infants and pregnant women.

- Soft cheeses made from unpasteurized milk (e.g., brie, Camembert, Roquefort, blue-veined, feta, queso blanco, queso fresco). Instead, eat hard cheeses such as cheddar or Swiss cheese. Read the product label to determine if the cheese was made using pasteurized milk.

- Raw or undercooked fish (such as sushi or sashimi)

- Refrigerated smoked seafood (such as tuna, mackerel, salmon, trout, and kippers) from the refrigerated section of supermarkets, seafood shops, and delicatessens. Canned tuna, salmon, and other fish products can be eaten.

- Salads that are ready-made in supermarkets and other retail stores. Make your own salads at home after careful washing of the ingredients, and use good hygiene during preparation.

- Refrigerated pâté or meat spreads available in supermarkets and delicatessens. Foods not needing refrigeration such as canned or shelf-stable pâté and meat spreads are safe to eat, but they must be refrigerated immediately after you open them.

- All raw food from animal sources (e.g., beef, pork, and poultry) should be cooked well to a safe internal temperature. Avoid "rare" steaks, and if your chicken has retained a pink colour toward the bone, do not eat it.

- Hot dogs, luncheon meats, cold cuts, and other deli meats (e.g., bologna) or fermented or dry sausages. Ensure that ground meats such as hamburger patties are *very* well cooked at a high enough temperature.

When preparing food, try to avoid contamination and cross-contamination. Salad vegetables must be well washed. Studies have shown that when chicken meat is washed and cut up, there is a widespread distribution of contaminating bacteria in the general vicinity of the preparation of the chicken. Therefore, other food items should not be close to the preparation area, and thorough cleaning of the area is recommended before other food items are placed in the same area. Remember to clean kitchen utensils well between the preparation of different foods.

"MUM, I CAN HEAR YOU!"

Be careful of what you are saying during those last few months of pregnancy. Someone may be listening — and that "someone" could be the soon-to-be-born fœtus you are nurturing.

It is unlikely that the fœtus can distinguish individual words, but during the last three months of pregnancy, brain development reaches a stage at which the areas of the brain that process sound become active. Hearing the outside world from within the womb would be rather muffled. As cognitive neuropsychologist Eino Partanen of the University of Helsinki explains it, "If you put your hand over your mouth and speak, that's very similar to the situation the fœtus is in. You can hear the rhythm of speech, rhythm of music, and so on."

As early as 1988, a study suggested that newborn babies recognized the theme song from their mother's favourite TV soap opera. Later studies indicated that when babies were born, they were already familiarized to the sounds of the native language of their parents but found the vowel sounds of other languages to which they were exposed unfamiliar.

In August 2013, the *Proceedings of the National Academy of Sciences of the United States of America* published a study using new testing techniques that took confidence in the hearing ability of the developing fœtus within the womb to a new level. As Eino Partanen explained, "Once we learn a sound, if it is repeated to us often enough, we form a memory of it, which is activated when we hear the sound again." In practice, the mechanism of such a memory helps one recognize the sound and cadence in the learner's native language — a good reason why, within households where two separate languages are used by the parents, from babyhood a child should be exposed to both languages. Children soon come to separate the languages from their differing tonalities, vowel sounds, and cadence patterns. Starting this process early in childhood develops better bilingual skills than the introduction of a second language in later years.

During the last few months of pregnancy, researchers at The University of Helsinki gave mothers a recording including a made-up word with occasional variations in the middle syllable, interspersed with music. On average, by the time their babies were born, the babies would have heard the made-up word more than 25,000 times. Using EEG (electroencephalogram) sensors to record electrical signals within their brains after they were born, it was found that these infants' brains recognized the made-up word and its variations.

The recognition signals were strongest in those babies of the mothers who had played the recording most often. There was a "control" group of babies whose mothers had not been provided with the recording. The babies exposed to the recording while in the womb were also better able to detect differences in the syllables, such as vowel length, than were the "control" babies. It was apparent that the observed learning effect was generalized to other types of similar speech sounds not included in the training recording. Partanen concluded, "This leads us to believe that the fœtus can learn much more detailed information than we previously thought."

Therefore, it is now established that during the last trimester of pregnancy, the fœtus is able to receive sound from outside the womb. This brain development also allows the fœtus to distinguish differences in the sounds it hears, even in the speech within its environment.

Researchers have studied music in the context of development, too. In the earliest days, weeks, months, and years of life, everything a child experiences and learns contributes to the stimulation of millions of vital connections within the brain — and these, in turn, form the foundation for all future learning. Research suggests that classical music, with its complexity, repetitions, and patterns, stimulates the brain in a way that may enhance math and science learning. Classical music may soothe as well, calming newborns and helping them adjust to life outside the womb. One reason could be that the soothing rhythm of most classical music is similar to that of the mother's heartbeat that surrounds the child from the moment hearing begins in the womb.

Could there be a more wonderful start to life for your baby than for you to relax during the last three months of your pregnancy and listen — along with your soon-to-be-born baby — to soothing classical music? In the chapter "**Helping Baby's Brain Development**," I pointed out that by the last weeks of the second trimester, neuron production within the brain is essentially complete, and the generation of the supporting glial cells is in progress. The third trimester is a period of rapid brain development, when the already-formed neurons begin to form connections (the synaptic connections) and when "superfluous" neurons are pruned. Connectivity comes from "challenges" to the neurons from the body's environment to form those synaptic connections. Obviously, then, hearing from the womb on a frequent basis the classical music you enjoy helps your soon-to-be-born baby to commence the learning experience of life in a better way.

Also by This Author:

HOW TO CHOOSE A BABY FORMULA

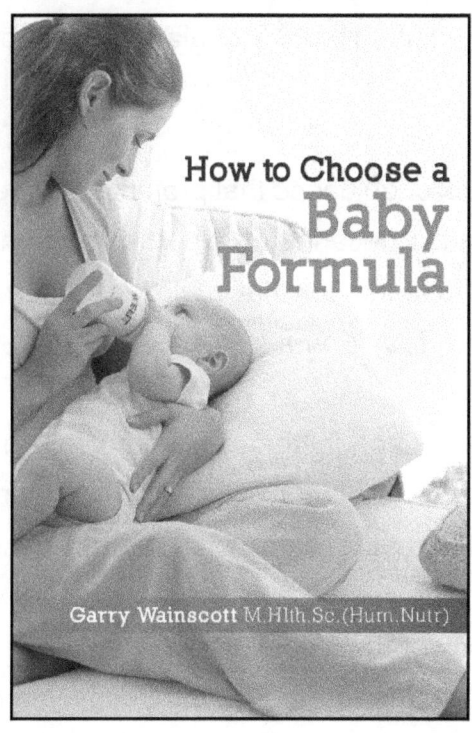

How many times has a mother been assisted greatly to begin and maintain breast-feeding, only to find at some later period that she has a need to supplement her breast-feeding with baby formula or is no longer able to continue breast-feeding and must turn to baby formula for adequate nutrition for her baby…only to find that there is no one to turn to for good advice in selecting the best baby for-mula for her baby?

Amazingly, little comprehensive and reliable information is available to a mother who finds herself in this situation to help her choose the most suitable formula for her baby's growth and development.

It was that lack of guidance that prompted the request to Garry Wainscott to put his decades of expertise and knowledge into a reliable, science-based book that could help these mothers. Thus, *How to Choose a Baby Formula* was born!

For example, although there is much talk out there about Omega-3, much of it is either misinformation or confusing. Garry's book goes into the real research to provide evidence-based infor-mation that explains the metabolism of Omega-3 within the body and the adequacy of the levels in baby formula required to make a significant difference to a baby's brain development. The book explains how to compare one baby formula with another when manufacturers use different value measurements on their labels.

And there is a whole lot more useful information in this book. To learn more about this book, go to www.babyformulachoice.com.

www.ingramcontent.com/pod-product-compliance
Lightning Source LLC
Chambersburg PA
CBHW051733170526
45167CB00002B/918